CAREER IN

ORTHOTICS

PROSTHETICS

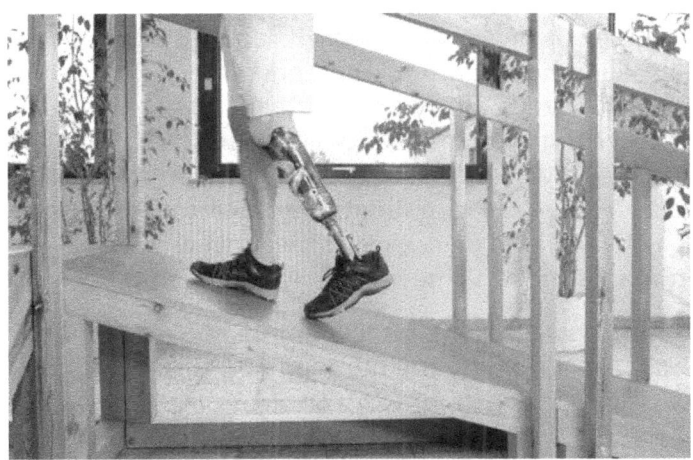

ORTHOTICS AND PROSTHETICS IS A unique component of the healthcare field that involves designing and fitting artificial limbs, braces, and other devices. Professionals in the field are often referred to as "O&P Practitioners." They work closely with people who have suffered from accidents, injuries, cancer, or other diseases, helping return them to an acceptable quality of life.

Although related, orthotics and prosthetics are not the same. Orthotics involves the design and fabrication of external braces (orthoses) as part of a patient's treatment process. The orthotic device helps control weakened or deformed regions of the body including the upper and lower limbs, cranium, or spine. The most common orthotic devices are back braces and shoe inserts needed to live a more comfortable life. Orthotic intervention can be life changing – or even lifesaving – for patients with scoliosis, severe neck injuries, or cerebral palsy.

Rather than supporting body parts, prosthetics involves replacing them. A prosthetist designs, creates, and fits artificial limbs on patients who are missing all or part of a limb. Creating a prosthesis requires a unique combination of art and technical skill. The prosthesis itself is much more complex than it may appear. It requires appropriate materials, alignment, design, and construction to match the functional needs of the individual that can vary greatly. Lower limb prostheses typically address stability in standing and walking, shock absorption, and aesthetics. In the case of patients who want to engage in athletic activities, the device must meet even more extraordinary functional needs.

Upper limb prostheses are no less complex. You do not know how extraordinary the human hand is until you no longer are able to reach, grasp, and manipulate objects. These devices can aid in the activities of daily living such as eating, dressing, and grooming. They can also be made to address specific occupational challenges such as hammering, painting, or writing.

A career in the field of prosthetics and orthotics can be very satisfying, both personally and professionally. Because of the work that orthotists and prosthetists do, patients who could not previously dance, lift everyday objects, or partake in the seemingly simple act of walking now have increased mobility and less pain.

The job outlook in this field is excellent! Job opportunities abound throughout the country, and the need for orthotic and prosthetic professionals is increasing rapidly. Nearly 30 percent of the current practitioners are over the age of 50 and will be entering retirement soon. As obesity, diabetes, and cardiovascular diseases continue to rise in America, there is more need than ever for people with this special skill set. Further, it is one of the few professions that can boast a 100 percent employment rate. Most people who enter the field choose to remain within it for life.

As an O&P professional you can make a difference every day! If you are interested in making a positive impact on people's lives, and entering a rapidly evolving unique health science career where the employment demand is exceptional, you may want to consider orthotics and prosthetics.

WHAT YOU CAN DO NOW

PREPARING FOR THIS CAREER IN HIGH SCHOOL starts with all available classes in math and science. Of particular importance are physics, biology, anatomy, and algebra, but all math and science are useful in this field. Also, look for any classes where you can tinker and work with your hands. Shop class, sculpture, or classes that involve robotics are ideal for improving your manual dexterity and the technical parts of your brain simultaneously (while building something cool in the process).

Join science clubs at school or in the community. If you are lucky, there will be a robotics club, but anything that involves the creation of 3-dimensional objects is a good choice.

Volunteer in your community. To better understand the kind of impact your potential career choice will have, spend some time with people who either have prosthetics or need them. Nursing homes and hospitals (especially VA hospitals) always need help. Being a volunteer will look good on a college application – and it might just change your life.

One of the best ways for you to get a taste of what it is like to work in this field is to "shadow" an orthotist in action. Job shadowing is a good idea no matter what career you are considering, but it is particularly valuable in the orthotics and prosthetics field. In fact, studies have shown that over 85 percent of students reported a positive change in their attitude towards this field after job shadowing. Ask your guidance counselor for help setting it up, or simply make your own introductory phone call to a local orthotist and express your interest. You will find that most of these professionals will be delighted to help.

HISTORY OF THE CAREER

Prosthetics

While those practicing today use some of the most advanced materials and technologies available, we can actually trace the field back thousands of years. Ancient peoples used rocks and branches to construct splints and braces for the injured and fashioned crude prostheses out of wood for amputees. Despite their primitive methods, they are the forefathers of today's practice, setting the healing stage for those wounded by accidents, battle, or disease.

There is evidence of prosthetics being used as far back as ancient Egypt. Historians have assumed that because these prostheses were crude, made of strong fibers and natural materials, the prostheses were mostly intended for form rather than function. They made the wearers "feel whole" once again, even though the devices were likely of no practical use. There have been some cases of ancient prostheses being functional – at least on a very small scale – like the female mummy who was discovered to have been given a new wooden toe when she was alive.

The years of ancient Rome also produced examples of prostheses, including an artificial leg made out of iron, bronze, and wood dating back to 300 BC. Other prostheses sightings are found in literature. For example, Herodotus spoke of a Persian who escaped his sentence of death by cutting off his own foot and building a replacement out of wood so he could walk to a nearby town. Another long ago writer, Pliny the Elder, told the tale of a Roman general who replaced a right arm lost in battle with an iron hand so he could mount his horse and ride once again.

In Medieval times, prostheses were constructed to hide deformities, particularly for those fighting in war. This allowed soldiers who had been wounded, to ride horses, hold shields, and generally keep up appearances after losing limbs. Because the devices were most often made of iron, they were incredibly heavy, which certainly must have limited their functionality. For those not involved in battle, there was a rise in wooden peg legs and hooks for hands. These are most commonly associated with pirates, but that is merely folklore. Any member of a ship's crew would want to remain useful and employed after an amputation. Made from the materials that could easily be found on a ship, prosthetic limbs were used to replace the ones lost by the crew. The ship's cook instead of a doctor trained in the field most often performed amputations on the high seas.

This period also saw some technical advancements in the construction of limbs. When some watchmakers started adding gears and springs, it represented a turning point in the history of prosthetics. It was considered a great triumph when a German mercenary named Gotz von Berlichingen ordered a pair of new iron hands in 1508. The hands were held on by leather straps. Because of their construction, springs allowed for actual movement of the prostheses, which had not been seen before.

The father of the modern form of amputation surgery, and prosthetics, as we know them today, is a Frenchman named Ambroise Paré. Paré is responsible for surgical techniques and new designs in prostheses for upper-extremity and lower-extremity amputees. He also advanced the engineering of these pieces by introducing things like fixed positions, adjustable parts, and locking control. Around this time, another Frenchman advanced the field by changing the prosthetic materials from a heavier iron to a much lighter combination of paper, glue, and leather. A Dutchman named Pieter Verduyn also invented a prosthesis for the lower leg constructed with hinges and leather. What each of these three men contributed to the field can still be seen in the modern prosthetics we know and use today.

During the 17th through 19th centuries, improvements came along swiftly, one after the other. There was Doctor Bly's anatomical leg in 1858, which he called the "most complete and successful invention ever attained in artificial limbs." There was suction technology, the first aluminum artificial limb, the Anglesey leg, and the first non-locking below-knee prosthesis. There were also advancements in amputation, such as a technique for ankle amputation that allowed patients to keep most of their lower appendage. Many of these advances came as the result of the Civil War, which was known for producing a huge number of amputees.

Anesthesia and better hygiene practices also moved amputation surgery closer to its current point, allowing doctors to perform for longer periods of time and with higher success rates. This meant that for the first time they could better control what the healed limb would look like, in effect pre-fitting it for the prosthesis that would take its place later.

In 1945, the National Academy of Sciences established the Artific al Limb Program to help meet the demand of the number of World War II veterans who returned home having left pieces of themselves back on foreign battlefields. Around this time, the polio epidemic also took place in the United States, resulting in many of America's children needing braces to walk.

The latter half of the 20th century saw the introduction of research programs into human locomotion, biomechanics, and technology that could benefit prosthetic development. As the field advanced, it also became apparent that there was a need to educate people, and the American Medical Association created a specialized certification for professionals in this field.

Today's prosthetics are made to move with their own microprocessors, chips, and robotics, bringing devices up to a level of functionality it has never before seen. In fact, some of these advancements sound like something out of a sci-fi movie. Take for example targeted muscle reinnervation, a procedure developed in Chicago by Dr. Todd Kuiken. Dr. Kuiken's surgery allows a doctor to reattach amputated nerves to a different, healthy muscle in the musculoskeletal system, thus allowing that nerve to function in a normal capacity. Instead of firing off signals into nowhere, however, it now fires them into the secondary muscle. The electrical charge that results can then be directed and used to control prosthetic limbs.

Orthotics

Orthotics can be traced back 2000 years to simple layers of wool that were added as a cushion in shoes to provide relief to the walker. In 1865, a man named Everett

Dunbar was the first on record to insert leather lifts into shoes, designed to support the foot's arches. Royal Whitman in Boston invented the first complete foot orthotic in 1905. The original design was actually quite a burden to its wearer, being heavy, clunky, and distorting their shoes. It did pave the way for a lighter and more functional version.

Dr. William Scholl, the most famous orthotist of all time, invented his first arch support device, known as the Foot-Easer, in 1910. When people saw how successful he was, there was actually a rush to get more orthotics on the market. False claims were made, advertisers lied, and in the 1940s the Federal Trade Commission decided something had to be done. They issued cease and desist orders, and orthotics took a major dip.

In the 1970s, jogging became a phenomenon, and suddenly everyone was complaining about shin splints and arch strains, resulting in new orthotics methods – this time with much lighter materials. Running shoes saw complete redesigns, now with built-in orthotics technology that supports the arch and adds a layer of cushion for runners.

WHERE YOU WILL WORK

SOME OF THE BIGGEST EMPLOYERS for orthotists and prosthetists include private physicians' practices, hospitals, rehabilitation centers, specialty clinics, home healthcare agencies, and nursing homes. Many also work in the laboratories of manufacturing facilities where these devices are made, modified or repaired.

Orthotists and prosthetists generally work in either an office or manufacturing setting. This is dependent on their individual specialty and the type of work they enjoy doing. However, of the 8,500 jobs in the orthotics and prosthetics field, most are situated in an office environment. Where that might be exactly, depends on the specific job role. Some orthotists and prosthetists work in private group practices, meeting with patients one on one to create perfect, customized solutions. About 10 percent work in a private physician's office. Others work in state, local, or private hospitals, where they often build more long-term, personal relationships with their patients.

The largest single group of orthotics and prosthetics specialists work in medical equipment and supplies manufacturing. That covers about 30 percent of all of those in the field. Health and specialty personal care stores are also employers, accounting for about a quarter of the workforce. The federal government employs another 10 percent of those in the field.

Most orthotists and prosthetists work full time and are at little risk for injury or illness in their jobs. It is a very safe field, at least for those who work in an office environment. Working in medical equipment and supplies manufacturing involves some risk, and precautions must be taken. To prevent injury from the materials and machines used to construct prosthetic devices, employees are often required to wear protective gear like goggles, gloves, and masks.

THE WORK YOU WILL DO

PROSTHETISTS AND ORTHOTISTS WORK closely with patients who have suffered from a debilitating injury, accident, or disease. Their goal is to help restore a patient's motion, function, and appearance. To do this, they may design medical supportive devices such as artificial limbs (arms, hands, legs, and feet), braces, and other medical or surgical devices. Each piece they produce is specifically designed to help the particular patient recover and live a happy, functional life.

There are numerous roles within this field, but the two main ones are prosthetists and orthotists.

Prosthetists work exclusively with patients who need a replacement limb. This can happen for a variety of reasons including birth defects, accidents and injuries, combat, cancer, or other diseases and conditions. They assess the patient, provide a treatment plan, order the prosthesis, demonstrate its use to the patient, and oversee the patient's recovery period.

Orthotists are more focused on areas like the spine or existing limbs that are malfunctioning or damaged. They work one-on-one with patients to solve these problems using equipment like braces and inserts.

Daily activities will differ depending on the job title and type of employer. However, all practitioners have the same or similar training, and many of the tasks overlap. Typically, orthotists and prosthetists do some or all of the following:

Evaluate and interview new patients to determine their needs

Take measurements to get the proper fit for the medical device

Make a mold of the patient's body part that will be fitted with a device

Select the materials to be used to make the device

Fit, test, and adjust devices on patients

Teach patients how to use their devices

Design orthopedic and prosthetic devices based on prescriptions from physicians

Repair or upgrade prosthetic and orthotic devices that have been used for a length of time

Keep detailed records of patient care and progress

General Orthotists and Prosthetists

The first thing that these practitioners do is get to know their patients and assess their current needs. This is done through a face-to-face meeting where they provide what is known as an "intake" examination. They may ask questions about the patient's history and then perform a series of small tests that determine the patient's current condition. Using their knowledge of kinesiology and biology, they note things like functional status, muscle development, sensory function, range of motion, joint stability, and skin integrity. Prosthetists will make measurements of the patient's residual limb, and orthotists will take measurements of the patient's affected area, or any part of the body needing treatment.

Getting a full understanding of a patient is key to developing a successful treatment plan. Each plan written by an orthotist or prosthetist is customized to the patient. Numerous factors are taken into account, including the patient's need for pain reduction, comfort level, stability, mobility, and desired aesthetics. Once the treatment plan is written, the practitioner reviews it with the patient, explaining how it will work, and what to expect. Patients typically have many questions, which will be answered at this time.

The next step in the process is to determine what might be the best device for the patient. It may be a brace, an insert, a lower extremity device, upper extremity device, or something else entirely. The selection is made based on the patient's needs as well as the specifications of the device itself – its durability, composition, and function. Price, availability, and insurance coverage may also be determining factors in the selection of the right prosthesis or orthotic for the particular patient.

The patient will then need to be prepared for the device. In order to do this, the practitioner will take precise measurements and casts, where appropriate, of the patient. The information will be used to write a prescription, which is sent along with the cast to the fabricator of the device.

CAD/CAM (Computer- Aided Design/Computer-Aided Manufacturing) technology is rapidly replacing the need for casting. With CAD/CAM, measurements can be scanned in by laser, or sometimes with a special hand-held wand. The collected information can describe the size and shape of the limb with utmost precision, allowing the practitioner to design a customized device for any patient entirely by using the computer. Once the design is finished, it can be downloaded to an automated carver that creates the actual orthotic or prosthetic device.

When the new device is delivered, the orthotist or pros-thetist will be responsible for checking the fit and comfort for the patient. It may be necessary to provide additions like compression garments or splints that will help the patient use the device and make the attachment more secure and comfortable. At this time, the practitioner will demonstrate its use and instruct the patient in how to take care of it.

The practitioner's job does not end when the patient leaves the office. The patient will need time to get used to using the device in everyday life. It is not uncommon for patients to experience discomfort. Sometimes it is temporary, but it can also mean there is an improper fit, and adjustment will be necessary. It can take weeks or even months to achieve the perfect fit for the patient. Throughout this process, the practitioner will carefully document the patient's progress in order to determine if the treatment plan is working effectively, or if changes need to be made.

Depending on the type and severity of the debilitation, a patient's recovery may require a team of healthcare providers, including therapists, physicians, nurses, dieticians, or physical therapists. In this case, the orthotist or prosthetist will interface regularly with these colleagues, working together as a team.

Orthotists or prosthetists who do not work in a clinical setting may find themselves with very different daily work activities. For example, they may work in a health or medical supply store. In this work setting, they will not likely develop such long-term relationships with their patients. Instead, they typically offer mostly pre-fabricated devices, or devices that leave a bit of room for customization, to patients who can use a more off-the-shelf option. They may also fill orders from other orthotists or prosthetists, taking charge of things like the stocking, pricing, inventory management, packaging, or shipping of devices to those who order them. They may also fill out paperwork or manage systems on the computer.

Some orthotists and prosthetists choose to supervise laboratories or manufacturing facilities. In this management capacity, they would oversee the facility's staff, making sure everything runs smoothly. They would assign projects and watch over their progress, ensuring all deadlines are met, and that team members are working in sync. They may order materials for the facility and stay on top of maintenance for any equipment.

Orthotists and prosthetists who run their own private offices will also need to deal with most of the same tasks, with a heavy emphasis on administrative and personnel duties. It will fall to them to ensure compliance with national standards and procedures, so they must stay on top of ever-changing laws and recommendations from authorities like the American Medical Association and Food and Drug Administration. They may hire someone to do this for them, but it is not always a cost-effective option.

Beyond the Generalist

Orthotists and prosthetists may also choose to enter a different aspect of the field altogether, getting away from handling patients and instead choosing to work in academia as a teacher or researcher. In roles like these, they may teach classes and train the next generation of prosthetists and orthotists, planning lessons, giving lectures, assigning and grading homework, or serving as a living textbook.

They may also lead their own teams, advancing the field further by delving deeply into new materials and technologies that can be used to make prosthetic or orthotic devices more lightweight, more intuitive, more comfortable, more affordable, more attractive, and more functional for the patients that need them.

Other common job titles in this field include:

Pedorthists – focus exclusively on the foot. They are

trained to assess lower limb anatomy, and their educational focus on biomechanics makes them especially qualified to make or modify corrective footwear. They use a unique set of tools to provide the appropriate shoes, shoe modifications, foot orthoses, and other devices.

Certified fitters – are highly trained in the specific area of the fit and delivery of prosthetic or orthotics devices. In particular, they work with prefabricated goods, which are not custom made for an individual patient. Some of these goods include orthotic fitters, breast prostheses, therapeutic shoes, or shoe inserts. They may work in a health and medical supply store filling orders or selling devices to patients or practitioners.

Certified technicians – are closely involved in the manufacturing and fit of the device, and not directly in the care of the patient. During a typical day, they may use equipment to modify a device, improve it for better fit or function, or change its aesthetics. In most cases these technicians are supervised by orthotists or prosthetists. They may also test devices for structure and stability before they are given to the patient. Technicians may work in a private laboratory, or they serve as an extension of a hospital and work for a team of doctors. Even though they do not interact one-on-one with patients, most certified technicians must stay on top of each patient's case so that they can easily make any changes as the patient's treatment plan unfolds.

Certified assistants – work closely with the orthotists and prosthetists in the area of patient care. They provide support for both the practitioners and the patients, answering questions and handling smaller pieces of the fabrication, modification or delivery of the prosthetic or orthotic. Certified assistants also help with the maintenance of the devices as well. They get to know their patients well, monitoring their progress and watching over their files.

STORIES OF PROFESSIONALS WORKING IN THE FIELD

I Specialize in Sports Prostheses

"It is an incredible feeling to have a person who entered my office in a wheelchair be able to walk out after being fitted with a new prosthesis. Helping an athlete is even more amazing. A good fitting orthosis or prosthesis helps them achieve their personal goals and fulfills their dreams. It also gives me a deep sense of satisfaction. I have worked with patients at every level, all the way up to members of the US Paralympic team. I have also traveled to many countries, demonstrating the latest techniques, and teaching others how to provide the highest quality care.

People who are unfamiliar with my profession may be unaware of the technological advances being made. Improved materials, some of which were originally developed for aerospace applications, are stronger and lighter than ever. Flexible polymers can eliminate any discomfort. Electronic knee joints can be programmed for each individual patient. A computer chip allows the knee joint to sense changes in position, speed, and force. That's what helps amputees walk down stairs and up hills. I also design prosthetic feet that are made for specific sports, such as running, golfing, or swimming. Upper limbs are even more amazing – able to detect complex electronic signals generated by muscles. These 'bionic arms' have the strength to swing a tennis racquet and the dexterity to pick up an egg.

The range of options available to O&P practitioners is practically unlimited. I'd advise anyone thinking about getting into the profession to contact a local practitioner and arrange a visit. You will see some of this cutting edge technology firsthand."

I Train People to Practice Pedorthics

"I owned a shoe repair shop when I first learned about pedorthics. Two orthopedic surgeons came into my shop and encouraged me to get some training in pedorthics. The need was (and still is) so great, they had decided to personally set out to recruit new people to the field. They were very persuasive, pointing out how I could make very significant improvements in peoples' lives. I got the training and have now owned a pedorthic company for more than 20 years. For the last 12 years, I have also been teaching pedorthics through community college courses and as a guest lecturer at many pedorthic schools around the country.

I treat patients of all ages who need help overcoming challenges related to diabetes, arthritis, and trauma. The work is personally very rewarding, and I would be very happy just working one-on-one with patients. But I also know that by teaching and training people to practice pedorthics, I can help many more people than my own client base. This is a wonderful profession, so diverse and so very much needed."

I Work With Veterans

"I am endlessly fascinated with the mechanical sciences, particularly as they apply to the human body. Orthotists like me build biomechanical devices that assist patients during rehabilitation by preventing, allowing, or restricting movement of a part of their body. Some patients will only need the device temporarily, while others will need it for their whole life.

I supervise the assignments of a staff of 25 O&P practitioners who work in a lab. We get our orders from three major military medical centers. My job is to coordinate the many technologies used for computer-assisted fabrication. Sometimes we still use older methods, such as negative casting to develop the device a physician has prescribed. But more often now, we will use a computer in a multi-step process that involves magnetic scanning, laser scanning, and photometric scanning, to create the image that will be sent to our 3D carver for fabrication.

We are in a time of rapid advances with new exciting tools and techniques introduced every day. One of the biggest improvements in the field is the invention of microprocessor knees. They are a miracle for anyone who has lost a leg above the knee. The prosthetic knee is programmed for the different phases of walking, such as heel strike, mid-stance, and push-off. The best part though, is that the microprocessor has a feature called 'stumble control' that prevents the wearer from falling.

The best thing about my work is that no two days are ever the same. Every day presents a different challenge, along with the opportunity to solve a different set of problems. What doesn't change is the end result and how it feels. There is nothing like seeing a young soldier who was previously in despair, but can now walk. He is the one with the ear-to-ear smile. I'm the one with the tear in my eye."

PERSONAL QUALIFICATIONS

WORKING IN ORTHOTICS AND PROSTHETICS requires a balanced mix of technical and interpersonal skills, backed by a deep-seated love for improving people's lives. Most experienced professionals in this field say that the more patients they serve, the stronger that combination becomes.

The most successful orthotists and prosthetists have many personal traits in common, such as natural talents for math and the sciences. This is a big advantage in a technical field that uses the principles of physics in the device's use, the foundation of chemistry in the device's construction, and precise measurements of mathematics in the device's design.

Another necessary trait is above-average manual dexterity. This is very detail-oriented work that requires shaping and measuring to create the perfect fit. Every patient's body is different – there is no such thing as a one-size-fits-all. It can take a few tries to get it right, and devices might need to be readjusted as people's bodies change. The easier time you have working with your hands, the faster and more accurate these changes will be for you.

Good communications skills will be needed as you interact with physicians, and patients and their families. For orthotists and prosthetists, asking the right questions and understanding the needs of patients are key parts of the work. After the prosthetic is made, they will also be explaining its use and care to the patients. This is an important part of the process. It must be articulated clearly and with patience, because very often this conversation has to be repeated more than once.

Sometimes patients require special, long-term care. In this case, you will need good interpersonal skills to develop a close working relationship. It starts with a caring demeanor and positive attitude. You will be part coach and part cheerleader. This is especially important as many patients who require prosthetic limbs have undergone some sort of major trauma, and may have a difficult time coming to terms with their new life. Because of their strong emotions, they may be a challenge to deal with, so they require a gentle bedside manner. Patients may also want to try many different types of prosthetics to find the one that works best for them. This can lengthen the process and require considerable patience.

Professionals in this field have a passion for what they do and are typically drawn to the work by the opportunity to help people. As an orthotist or prosthetist, you will be making a difference to your patients and their families on a daily basis. Because of the device you make, mobility is restored – and so is hope. Few careers have such a noticeable and direct impact on people. A strong desire to experience that will shine through in your work.

For those considering opening their own office, skills like organization, leadership, and time management become essential. You could be handling multiple patients simultaneously along with all of the day-to-day office management.

ATTRACTIVE FEATURES

A CAREER IN PROSTHETICS AND orthotics can be very rewarding. The devices you make for your patients allow them to feel better and heal. By using the latest technology to construct artificial limbs, your work allows patients to regain mobility and range of motion that they did not have before they met you. Imagine people walking into your office with severe mobility issues. Now imagine them leaving, knowing that they can now walk, jump, dance, or play. Experienced professionals in the field say that it is a privilege to be part of that kind of transformation.

If your patient lost a limb or other body part to cancer, injury or other disease, you might also produce something that makes your patient feel beautiful again or restore a long-lost feeling of being "normal." As such, many people find that being involved in the process of rehabilitating or reconstructing a patient gives them a personal feeling of joy in having given something back to the people they work with.

With the rapidly advancing technology in robotics and materials, it is a very exciting time to be a part of it all. If you love to learn, you will enjoy the educational opportunities. Part of your job will be keeping up with the latest technology, and staying on top of new releases of improved computer imaging, updated devices, microprocessors, and myoelectric joints.

Many people consider the high earnings potential and the growing demand in the field to be attractive features as well. The salary for an experienced professional is close to six figures. Some surpass that, and without the requirement of many years of expensive schooling.

The biggest advantage of choosing a career in orthotics or prosthetics is the excellent job outlook. Job opportunities are everywhere, and the growing need for new careerists is not expected to slow down in the foreseeable future. Every year, 125,000 Americans lose limbs due to diseases like cancer, advanced arthritis, Multiple Sclerosis, Parkinson's Disease, and diabetes. Many more have orthopedic impairments due to obesity, sports activities, birth defects, or traumas related to automobile accidents and military combat. There are millions of Americans counting on orthotists and prosthetists to help them. Many will find there is a shortage of these professionals, and they will not be able to get the help they need. This translates to job security, both for new graduates and for those already in the field. Those in the field stay because the work is so rewarding. In fact, nearly all professionals in this field make it their lifelong career.

UNATTRACTIVE ASPECTS

WHILE WORKING IN THE FIELD OF orthotics or prosthetics is quite emotionally rewarding, it can also be emotionally taxing. Professionals in this field see the impact of trauma on a daily basis. They work closely with car crash victims, veterans who have lost their limbs in combat, elderly patients who are struggling and find it very painful to walk, patients who have lost parts of their body to cancer and may still be fighting the disease, obese adults who have experienced amputations due to diabetes, babies with birth defects, and people who are battling all kinds of disabling conditions. These patients will have their good days and bad. When the going gets tough, you can expect tears, insults, anger, frustration, and tantrums. It is only human nature and certainly understandable, but dealing with it can be difficult.

Practitioners might also lose patients to a disease or condition. The longer you have served a patient, the harder it will be to handle your own personal emotional aftermath. You will need to remain strong and calm to deal with grieving families who have not only lost a loved one, but have to grapple with administrative issues such as paperwork, insurance, or payments. It is the worst that can happen, and it does not happen often, but it does happen in most healthcare professions.

In this field, there can be some very annoying bureaucracy. Things like negotiating with insurance companies and plowing through red tape can be a big part of the job for those working in hospitals or private practices. Some days it will seem like you will never get to the bottom of the mountain of paperwork. Those who work with veterans will face a huge volume of government forms and contracts that must be filled out for each patient.

There can also be a substantial amount of trial and error with patients while they get fitted for the right prosthetic or orthotic device. You must have endless patience. Your patients, on the other hand, often get impatient – and with good reason. It can be very time-consuming and frustrating for patients who have taken home multiple devices that failed to provide the relief that they sought, and who desperately want to move on with their lives. It can be frustrating for you, as well.

This is also a highly specialized field. While there is exceptional job security, and the demand for prosthetists and orthotists is high, it is not a career that can easily transition into other professions. To change careers would likely mean starting over completely. Fortunately, the work is so satisfying, most professionals do not want to change careers.

EDUCATION AND TRAINING

PEOPLE WHO WANT TO PURSUE A career in the area of prosthetics and orthotics can expect to spend between four and six years in college. Although there are a few different ways to train for this field, such as obtaining a bachelor's degree in orthotics and prosthetics, or completing a certificate program, master's degrees are becoming more and more important. In fact, the National Commission on Orthotics and Prosthetic Education has recommended that all bachelor's degree programs transition to master's degree programs as minimum preparation for this career.

There are still bachelor's programs that specialize in orthotics, prosthetics, or both. In four-year university settings, students can expect to take courses that are heavy in mathematics and the sciences. Subjects like biology, chemistry, physics, kinesiology, biochemistry, mathematics, psychology, and anatomy are emphasized. Before graduating, students will also be expected to complete general education requirements. Each school has its own rules on this, but expect that mathematics and science classes will need to be balanced by courses in communications, literature, and foreign language.

Students may also take clinical courses during this degree program and will likely be required to complete a senior capstone project. This is a two-semester process in which students pursue independent research on a question or problem of their choice. Under the guidance of a faculty mentor, they participate in scholarly debates in the relevant disciplines. To complete the project, they must also produce a substantial paper that confirms the student has a deep understanding of the topic.

It is not necessary to get a four-year degree specifically in orthotics or prosthetics to practice in this field. There is also the option of getting an undergraduate degree and then continuing with a master's. There are a number of undergraduate majors that can prepare students for a master's program in orthotics or prosthetics. Some of the best include engineering, kinesiology, biology, and bioengineering.

To qualify for admission into a master's program,

students must have at least a C average or higher, but this is dependent on the particular university's admissions requirements. Some universities require a 3.0 on a 4.0 scale, or they might only consider candidates who have taken certain classes in their undergraduate programs. It is important to research master's programs before applying, while still an undergraduate if possible.

The master's programs take a much more comprehensive approach to the field and involve activities such as clinical rotations, examinations, and laboratory work. Coursework is typically focused on the device side of the field, with classes such as plastics, or other materials. Classes can also include advanced science subjects such as neuroscience. Each master's program is different, but they typically require up to 500 hours of work in a clinical setting before students are allowed to graduate. People who graduate with master's degrees in this field are eligible for just about any position in the field, including academia and research.

Certification

To obtain certification, applicants must enroll in a one-year program that focuses on clinical education. The Commission on Accreditation of Allied Health Education Programs is the body responsible for the accreditation of these programs. The programs allow students to aim for certification in either orthotics or prosthetics, though some practitioners choose to be certified in both in order to advance their career prospects. To gain admittance, applicants are expected to have a bachelor's degree with an emphasis in math and the sciences. In particular, students should have completed courses in biology, chemistry, physics, psychology, math, human anatomy, and physiology.

Practitioners are also required to compete a one-year

residency program under a licensed professional before they can strike out on their own. The National Commission on Orthotic and Prosthetic Education keeps a list of approved residency programs. Upon completing the residency, the new practitioners may sit for the American Board for Certification in Orthotics, Prosthetics and Pedorthics examination. Not every state requires this, but most orthotists and prosthetists are certified through this examination. Once applicants pass the certification exam, they will be designated as Certified Orthotists, Certified Prosthetists, or Certified Prosthetists/Orthotists.

EARNINGS

THE SALARY RANGE FOR AN ORTHOTIST or prosthetist can vary widely depending on multiple factors such as geographic location and type of employer. Generally, the more experienced and specialized you are, the more you can expect to make in this field. Overall, the average annual salary is about $65,000 nationwide. The lowest paid make less than $40,000 per year. Those in the top earnings category clear three times as much, or about $115,000 on average. It takes time and experience to reach that salary level – 15 years in the field seems to be the threshold to rise above six figures in income.

Entry-level salaries for orthotists and prosthetists start at a respectable $35,000. That is for new residents just starting out in the first year after completing their National Commission on Orthotic and Prosthetic Education (NOPE). Most of these professionals stay in the profession for their entire working lives. As each year passes, their annual salary has the potential to grow by thousands of dollars. Those with an average of 15 years of experience earn an average compensation (base salary plus any bonus and commissions) of just over $95,000, according to a recent professional survey. Other salaries in the report include:

Certified pedorthist with an average or 15 years of experience
$60,000

Certified technician with an average of 15 years of experience
$55,000

Certified assistant with an average of six years of experience
$50,000

Certified fitter with an average of seven years of experience
$45,000

How much orthotists and prosthetists earn also depends on the particular employment situation The top five highest-paying fields are:

Medical equipment and supplies manufacturing

Health and personal care stores

Federal government

Office settings

General medical and private practice hospitals

Those working in the medical equipment and supplies manufacturing sector earn an average $70,000 per year, while their counterparts in health and personal care stores earn slightly less, just under $65,000. Federal government workers are also in that salary range, with an average salary of $65,000 per year. Those in private practice office settings earn less, only $55,000. The average salary for those in more general medical offices, including group practices and hospitals is about $50,000.

OPPORTUNITIES

RECENT REPORTS POINT TO MORE than 5,500 orthotists and prosthetists practicing today. Of these, about 35 percent are certified orthotists, 25 percent are certified prosthetists, and 40 percent are certified in both. It is a great time to join this field, with an expected employment expansion rate of over 35 percent during the coming decade. That translates to about 3,000 new jobs.

The national healthcare crisis has created a very high demand for specialists in orthotics and prosthetics. Aging baby boomers and an increase in cases of obesity and diabetes in America are setting the stage for more people than ever who need prosthetic limbs or orthotic care. There are simply too few people trained and qualified to provide services. The US Department of Education has even made a public call for more people to enter the field, saying that training in this industry is a "national priority with a practitioner deficit." Attrition is not helping the situation either. In fact, it is widening the gap even further. Nearly 30 percent of current practitioners who are certified in both prosthetics and orthotics are set to retire in the next 10 years. The same goes for certified pedorthists.

The National Health Interview Survey reported that one in eight Americans have disabling conditions that interfere with life activities, and 16 percent of those individuals reported an orthopedic impairment. Currently, more than 3.5 million Americans use orthotics or braces because of diseases or conditions that cripple or disable. That number is expected to grow exponentially over the next

20 years.

The Department of Health and Human Services calls diabetes and obesity the "twin epidemics." Diabetes is the number one cause of limb loss today, and by 2020, 35 million Americans are expected to have the disease. This will dramatically increase the number of prosthetics needed. The second leading cause of amputation is vascular problems among the elderly and obese. Vascular reconstruction can utilize lighter materials than ever before, making it possible for prosthetics to be used where they might not have worked in the past. The technology is outpacing the number of educated prosthetists available to work with these patients.

It is not just patients with diseases who require the sort of care that only an orthotist or prosthetist can provide. Sufferers from car crashes, sports injuries, combat, birth defects, and many other types of accidents also create a nonstop need for services. There simply are not enough people entering the field to take care of all of these patients. If the current trend continues, by 2020, two-thirds of the people needing orthotic care or prosthetics will not be able to have their needs met. That is millions of people lacking adequate care.

Exciting new materials, advancing technology, and the prolonging of life also contribute to the increased opportunities within this field.

GETTING STARTED

YOU HAVE COMPLETED YOUR EDUCATION and you are ready to search for your first job. Here is some great news: graduates in this field have a 100 percent employment rate. Few careers can match that! What you need to consider is the type of job you want and where you want to work.

Does medical equipment and supplies manufacturing sound appealing to you? If so, make a list of potential employers. If you like interacting more closely with the public, a health or personal care store could be a better fit for you. You might also consider a job in the federal government or office setting. If you are the type of person who enjoys working one-on-one with patients and getting to know them on a long-term basis, a general medical hospital or private practice could be a great place for you to start.

Once you have decided where you would like to work, you will need to send them your résumé. Because this is your first job, most of the information on your résumé will be the classes you took throughout college, especially the ones that are most relevant to the career path you are pursuing. Also, include any organizations you have joined, as well as extra certifications you have received. Volunteer positions and internships carry some weight. In fact, any work you have done in the field – paid or unpaid – is valuable experience that should be included.

To find job openings, start at your school's career center or job placement office. They will also provide help with résumé and cover letter writing, mock interviews, and follow-up techniques. Your career counselor can also hook you up with recruiters.

Network with your professors and peers. Make sure everyone knows what you are looking for and how to reach you if they should hear of an opening. By now, you should have joined at least one professional organization. Look for others that you can join. If you want to work where you are living, start participating actively at the local level. It is the fastest way to learn about who is hiring. If you want to work elsewhere or do not mind relocating for the right position, make regular visits to the websites of professional organizations. There you will find job postings as well as events scheduled around the country where you can meet people face to face.

Not everyone will be recruited the day they graduate, but persistence pays off in job searching. The more people you meet and the more feelers you put out there, the more likely you will find the perfect position for you.

ASSOCIATIONS

■ **American Orthotic Prosthetic Association**
http://www.aopanet.org

■ **American Academy of Orthotists and Prosthetists**
http://www.oandp.org

■ **American Board for Certification in Orthotics, Prosthetics & Pedorthics (ABC)**
https://www.abcop.org

■ **National Association for the Advancement of Orthotics and Prosthetics**
http://www.naaop.org

■ **National Commission on Orthotic and Prosthetic Education (NCOPE)**
http://www.ncope.org

PERIODICAL

■ **Journal of Orthotics and Prosthetics**
http://www.oandp.org/jpo

WEBSITES

■ **OP Careers**
http://www.opcareers.org

■ **OandPCare.org**
http://www.oandpcare.org

www.ingramcontent.com/pod-product-compliance
Lightning Source LLC
Chambersburg PA
CBHW070753180526
45168CB00004B/1599